WHEN YOU ARE COPING

DIFFICULT TIMES SERIES

WHEN YOU ARE COPING WITH INFERTILITY

VERA SNOW

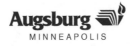

Augsburg
MINNEAPOLIS

*This book is dedicated to my daughters, Gracie
and Isabel, and especially to my husband, Greg.*

WHEN YOU ARE COPING WITH INFERTILITY

Copyright © 2002 Augsburg Fortress. All rights reserved. Except for
brief quotations in critical articles or reviews, no part of this book
may be reproduced in any manner without prior written permission
from the publisher. Write to: Permissions, Augsburg Fortress, Box
1209, Minneapolis, MN 55440.

Large-quantity purchases or custom editions of this book are available at a discount from the publisher. For more information, contact
the sales department at Augsburg Fortress, Publishers, 1-800-328-
4648, or write to: Sales Director, Augsburg Fortress, Publishers, P.O.
Box 1209, Minneapolis, MN 55440-1209.

Cover Design by David Meyer
Book Design by Jessica A. Klein

Library of Congress Cataloging-in-Publication Data
Snow, Vera, 1967-
    When you are coping with infertility / Vera Snow.
        p.cm.
    ISBN 0-8066-4360-9 (alk. paper)
    1. Infertility—Psychological aspects. I. Title.
RC889.S59 2002
616.6'92'0019—dc21   2001045806

The paper used in this publication meets the minimum require-
ments of American National Standard for Information Sciences—
Permanence of Paper for Printed Library Materials, ANSI
Z329.48-1984. ♾ ™

Manufactured in the U.S.A.   AF 9-4360

06   05   04   03   02   1   2   3   4   5   6   7   8   9   10

❧ Contents ❧

❧ *Introduction* ❧

Infertility is a complex condition that only gets more complicated as you continue to learn about it. The experience of this condition can be a long and arduous journey—physically, emotionally, and spiritually. As with any demanding journey, it is important to treat yourself gently, no matter how frustrated or frightened you might become. It is important to surround yourself with people who will provide strength and understanding even when nothing seems to make sense to you. This is a difficult time in your life, one in which your pain and feelings should be respected and validated, first by yourself and then by others.

This book will not tell you what decisions to make about your medical options. You will not be told what is right or wrong. You will, however, receive guidelines to help you focus and use your energy wisely. You will find suggestions on how to optimize your actions toward resolution and wholeness, as well as how to distinguish that which is out of your control. I will apply recognized descriptions of the grief and loss cycle to the infertility experience and help you discover ways to take care of yourself, establish support systems, explore your options, and seek resolution.

Essentially, this book offers comfort and encouragement as you cope with infertility and struggle for personal understanding of a medically challenging condition that has personal ramifications that often touch the core—self-image, self-esteem, and self-understanding. I write from the perspective of one who has gone through it. I have also worked with others along the way and hope our combined experience will shed light on this difficult time for you as well.

⊷ Chapter One ⊷

Admitting Your Powerlessness

After many months of trying to conceive a child, I found it hard to accept that my husband and I had not succeeded. Nothing could have prepared Greg and me for the experiences that lay ahead once we placed ourselves in the hands of medical professionals whose specialty was infertility. We were suddenly faced with so many choices: Which procedure should we try? Should we use more aggressive medications? Will a different doctor bring better results? Nothing seemed to work, and it seemed that the harder we tried, the worse it got.

Our marriage was put to the test—many tests, in fact. Reproduction is a fundamental aspect of human life and marriage. When a couple that wants children is faced with the prospect of not having any, the stress can be severe. We spent much of our time crying, arguing, praying, and attempting to come up with solutions. I have often remarked, since then, that if we could make it through infertility we could make it through anything. There is probably more truth to that than even I realize.

THE BATTLE FOR CONTROL

Infertility is a medical condition that makes you realize quickly how little control you have over the situation. As soon as you choose to confront this condition, you are inundated with unknowns and uncertainties. First, you and your spouse go through a series of tests to find out what's wrong. Sometimes the doctors can make a diagnosis, but sometimes they cannot. Sometimes they can present a prognosis, sometimes they cannot. You inevitably become immersed in a medical subculture in which you hear story after story of couples who have tried every infertility procedure known to science, only to conceive after giving up and stopping all treatments. You witness highly skilled doctors who become consistently humbled by projecting a couple's chances for attaining pregnancy and finding out they are completely off the mark. If there is an underlying message that comes through this subculture, it is that infertility is beyond our control. No matter what the statistics say or what you expect to happen, infertility continues to baffle the couples who are trying to overcome it and the medical personnel who try to help them.

During our experience with infertility, my husband and I constantly battled for control and could have easily been lured into a sort of infertility addiction. Getting pregnant became an obsession. I had trouble letting go and admitting my powerlessness. I thought the trick to getting pregnant was to be diligent and hard-working. This seemed to work in other life situations, so why shouldn't it now? I decided to put all my efforts into becoming the perfect patient. I took my medications regularly and did everything I was told by my doctors. But nothing happened. Every month presented the same series of dilemmas: Should we try one more round of treatments or save our money for adoption? Should we work on both at the same time? When I finally began to admit my power-lessness, however, I found myself moving forward toward resolution.

In our "you can have it all" society, conceiving children is often perceived as something to which, if and when we want it, we are entitled. It's just one more thing we can work to achieve, like home own-ership or financial success. And like anything else we might try to achieve, we are faced with many choices—in the case of infertility treatments, more choices than ever before. It is easy to conclude that having more options means having more control. But conceiving a child, as a fundamental element of human life and identity, is unlike other forms of achievement. Faced with so many choices, it is easy to become overwhelmed, anxious, and desperate. For many, life seems to spiral out of control during the infertility experience. At some point—and this point will arrive differently for each couple and even each spouse—it is important to recognize that you cannot be in control of everything.

*F*INDING BALANCE

Finding balance is key to coping with infertility. In this case, balance means to decipher what you can and cannot control. No matter how your infertility is resolved—through conception and birth, adoption, or acceptance of life without children—recognizing your limits is the first step toward healing. Knowing when to let go and when to let God is the next step. It is difficult to maintain this balance, but learning to find it is a skill you will value for the rest of your life.

How do you surrender power and control? This can be different for everyone. Basically, however, it means surrendering to something bigger than yourself. It means acknowledging that you don't have all the answers. Thinking in this manner may lead to prayerfulness or some kind of personal ritual for inviting grace and guidance. But by admitting your powerlessness over infertility, it becomes significantly easier to bear the burden. You become able to concentrate on what you do have control over, and let the rest go. With limited responsibility, you can optimize your efforts. Whatever the ultimate outcome of your struggle with infertility, you can focus your energy on healing and wholeness.

❧ Chapter Two ❧

Recognizing the Loss
and Grief Cycle

My first experience with loss and grief came at nineteen when my mother died of ovarian cancer. At the time, I didn't know anything about the loss and grief cycle. I had no idea if my misery would ever come to an end. Many years later, when infertility came into my life, I found myself better equipped to move through the grieving process.

Grief is an essential part of infertility. It is not an option or a subtle side-effect. You are dealing with the loss of a dream, loss of privacy, loss of control, and sometimes, even loss of a life. Often the sense of loss will be a part of you for a long time, even after your infertility is resolved—sometimes forever.

The first thing to remember about grief is that it manifests itself differently in each person and in each situation. Even though grief is unpredictable in many ways, it still must be worked through. Attempting to squash, avoid, or short-circuit the grieving cycle will not be effective. Accepting grief can be quite liberating, especially when you are busy trying to control other factors in your life.

The key is to put all your losses into perspective and empower yourself to see the grief cycle through in its entirety. Your energy will be much better spent on understanding the cycle and preparing for ways to get through it, rather than in trying to keep it from happening.

THE STAGES OF LOSS AND GRIEF

In her book *On Death and Dying*, Elisabeth Kübler-Ross defines the five stages of death. These stages are commonly used to describe the grieving cycle as well. Because infertility is comprised of one loss after the other, understanding these five stages can be quite helpful.

Denial/Isolation

This first stage usually comes in the form of the statement, "No, not me." It may occur during the initial infertility diagnosis or may return on a monthly basis. Getting your period may trigger a denial reaction and force you and your spouse into solitude. The last thing you want to face are inquiring minds who ask, "Is there any news this month?"

Anger/Resentment

In this stage we pose the question, "Why me?" Denial passes and may be replaced by feelings of anger, rage, and resentment. Anger is manifest in various ways, and is sometimes directed toward others. For instance, if you surround yourself with the support of other couples who are also experiencing infertility, you may be caught off guard when one of those couples becomes pregnant. Your happiness for them may be tainted by feelings of anger and envy. You may also find yourself blaming doctors, clinics, and God.

Fear/Bargaining with God

In the third stage, we aim to postpone the inevitable by entering into some sort of agreement. This usually includes a promise to not ask for anything more if only this one wish would come true.

Sadness/Depression

During this stage we express sorrow over our circumstances. No amount of cheering up or looking on the bright side of things will suffice. If one spouse is more optimistic or upbeat one month, it is important that the other spouse be respected and acknowledged for his or her negative feelings as they occur. If sadness is what he or she is feeling, this needs to be experienced and expressed before acceptance can happen.

Acceptance

Kübler-Ross describes this stage as a form of quiet expectation. It follows the mourning process when all feelings have had the opportunity to be expressed. Acceptance should not be mistaken for happiness, it is rather a period of rest. During infertility, acceptance can occur every month as each cycle presents an end as well as hope for the future. This is the stage that gives infertility the feeling of a roller coaster ride. When you've finally accepted the empty result of one cycle, your hopes are already on the rise for the next one. The acceptance stage may accompany the final resolution of infertility as well.

❧

These stages become part of the monthly drill. By the time you have accepted one month's "failure," you become hopeful again for the next month. Before you know it, you are gearing up for another potential grief cycle to take place. Eventually, it might be hard to keep up with this roller coaster ride of emotions, and you might become stuck in sadness and depression. Try to avoid emotional stagnation by recognizing the stages and giving each the time needed to be worked through.

*T*HE TEST OF TIME

Ironically, time, the most common healing factor, can work against you during infertility. Time becomes a monster on your back and a constant reminder of how long you have waited for a baby. You may begin to believe that life is measured in monthly increments with nothing but empty space in between. Attentiveness to the grieving process can help you overcome the negative impact of time in this case.

During my fertility treatments, I made many trips to the drug store to buy pregnancy test kits. On a good day, I even teased myself about buying stock in them. I couldn't wait an entire week after missing a menstrual cycle (as recommended on the package) and took my first test after the first day of missing my period. While waiting for the result, I would squint my eyes and hold it up to the light so as not to miss the first hint of blue color, should it appear. If the test came out negative, I would discard the result as "too early" and pray my bleeding wouldn't start the next day. Eventually, each negative result became too hard to take, and I finally had to stop taking pregnancy tests altogether. It was easier to pretend that I might be pregnant than to risk finding out that I wasn't.

Denying the truth was a significant part of my monthly grieving cycle. Of course, not everyone becomes obsessed with pregnancy tests. Everyone experiences grief differently. It is not helpful to compare yourself to others. Some stages last longer, while others go by quickly. Unfortunately, it takes time and patience to grieve, which is incompatible with the ticking clock of infertility. Give yourself a break and accept the grieving process as a necessary part of the healing process. No amount of willpower can speed things up. Sometimes expressing it and putting it into words is a way to get through it:

Dear God,

I got my period today.

This marks another cycle of failure.

We have to wait another whole month to try and make a baby.

To us, thirty days seems like an eternity.

Please help us to endure the days ahead.

Steer us away from living in the future and keep us focused on today.

We hand over our anxiety and thoughts of hope-
lessness in exchange for the gift of patience.
Amen

Resolving Grief

After my mother died, I did everything I could to
keep going. I was young, in college, and supposed to
be having the time of my life. At the age of nineteen,
grieving was not on the top of my priority list, so I
filled my time with other things. When I reached
adulthood, my unresolved grief became stifling.
Grief eventually overwhelmed my system, and I got
stuck in a deep depression. I decided to seek help. My
counselor told me that I was using more energy to
stifle the grieving process than I would if I would just
let it take its course. Because my depression became
clinical, I was given an antidepressant in conjunction
with cognitive therapy. I was then able to emote and
work through a grief that was long past due.

For a patient who is also in the midst of infertility treatments, however, clinical depression is hard to
tackle. Antidepressants are prohibited because of the
detrimental effects they might have on a fetus. There-
fore, it becomes especially important to pay attention
to the grieving cycle. Try not to stifle the grief; find
ways to let it flow. Give yourself opportunities to
emote by listening to sad music or renting a tear-
jerker video. Take up kick-boxing to encourage physical and emotional release. Start practicing yoga to
strengthen your nervous system and increase your
stress resistance.

Whatever you decide to do, remember that you can have a proactive role in allowing the grief cycle to run its course toward healing. Focus your energies where they will be most productive. Concentrate on becoming aware of what your body and mind are telling you. Look beyond ways to "medicate and avoid." Distractions might be helpful and necessary at times, but shouldn't become routine. Steer clear, for example, of throwing yourself into your work or seeking overtime at the office. And most importantly, do not pretend that things are normal, because they are not. This will only prolong the grieving process by keeping you in the denial stage.

The point is to try to become aware of how you are or are not dealing with your grief. This is where your responsibilities lay. The grief itself will take its own form and will come and go in its own way. Your job is to help yourself prepare and provide healthy ways for the grief to express itself. This, of course, is easier said than done—but it must be done.

❧ Chapter Three ❧

Discovering How to Take Care of Yourself

When my husband and I first realized that we were having trouble conceiving a child, we were quick to confide in an array of people. Then, when a friend gave me a stack of information on adoption, I became hysterical. I wept at the notion that our infertility was irreversible. We were newly diagnosed with infertility and were in the preliminary stages of looking at treatment plans, and my friend thought it would be appropriate to bombard us with adoption information. Though adoption eventually became the perfect resolution for us, we were not ready to face that decision at that particular time. We needed people to listen and acknowledge our struggle. We didn't need unsolicited advice.

SET BOUNDARIES

One of the first things you learn when battling infertility is that people instinctively want to help with your situation. They mean well, but may unknowingly make comments that are demeaning and patronizing. They say: "Just relax and let nature take its course" or "The minute you decide to adopt, you will become pregnant" or "God must have a special plan for you." Ironically, "helpful" comments such as these do the opposite of what they are intended to do.

They often provoke feelings of anger, guilt, and shame that make it difficult to deal with the true emotions that lie just below the surface. You should never have to doubt your feelings, especially not in the midst of crisis. Infertility can make you feel as if your world is falling apart. Being subjected to comments implying that it's "no big deal" is detrimental to your healing process. Infertility causes many wounds that deserve to be given time to heal. It's your responsibility to make sure these wounds are protected. Setting boundaries is a key to taking care of yourself.

How do you set boundaries? Begin by being discriminating about who you do and do not tell about your infertility. Some people have an especially supportive family or community of friends while others may only have a few people in whom to confide. It is completely up to you to decide to whom and how much or how little you want to divulge. Remember, infertility is a big deal and piggy-backs on bigger issues. For instance, some women begin to question the meaning of womanhood in their lives. Men may face issues pertaining to the continuation of their name and blood line. For others, it's the loss of a dream or a significant glitch in the natural progression of a marriage. With an issue so multi-layered, it is important to take care about the number and character of one's confidants.

I talked with a woman who told some inquiring co-workers, "Nothing new, but you will be the first to know when I have something to share." This is a tactful way of telling someone they are important to you, but also letting them know that you don't want your whole relationship with them to revolve around infertility. It's easy to forget that people who truly care about you will find great pleasure in seeing you taking care of yourself. They will embrace the idea of you claiming responsibility for your well-being. Sometimes it's hard to believe, but the last thing they want to do is add more frustration to your life.

*P*UTTING YOURSELF FIRST

We often leave taking care of ourselves on the back burner. Feelings of guilt and selfishness are frequently associated with self care. It seems easier to take care of everything and everyone else first. You may feel pressure to keep moving along at the same pace and discount the fact that your energy level is different these days. What seemed like a manageable schedule before may now be significantly more difficult because you aren't compensating for the extra physical and emotional challenges you are facing.

You may need to change your priorities for the time being. What seemed important and essential at one time may not seem so important now that infertility has entered the picture. Here again, you have to decide what is within and what is outside of your control. Taking care of yourself has to become a top priority and a responsibility you need to own. How you put that responsibility into action is completely up to you.

REMEMBER YOUR PHYSICAL WELL-BEING

While it is important to address your emotional well-being, it is also important to concentrate on your physical health as well. Paying attention to both and seeing how they correlate to each other can bring you to an optimum state for healing. Movement is a great way to keep your head clear and move the energy around in your body. Some people find exercise to be meditative, a way to get in touch with something bigger than yourself, while also physically relieving the body of stress.

I had an epiphany once while on the treadmill. The monotonous motion kept me in rhythm with my breath, and I somehow got in touch with the twenty-third Psalm. I was internally chanting, "The Lord is my Shepherd, I shall not want," and was overcome by a sense of peace. Suddenly, I became aware of my own journey through the valley of darkness and admitted that infertility was indeed a crisis for my life. I also became aware that I wasn't alone, and that this, too, would pass. This moment in the gym gave me a spark of hope that I didn't have before. It opened me up to the idea that infertility was a significant part of my life-journey and would resolve itself in its own time and in its own way.

LETTING GO, AGAIN

If letting go and letting God is one way of coping with infertility, where does that leave you? It invites you to keep life simple. It asks you to take things one day at a time. Instead of living for the end of each menstrual cycle, try living one moment at a time. This may entail hot bubble baths at the end of the day, renting videos with your partner on weeknights, reading other people's memoirs, or going for long walks with your dog. It means listening to soothing music in a traffic jam, reading inspirational books before bed, or just journaling to unscramble your thoughts and feelings. Basically, it means treating yourself carefully and nurturing yourself from the inside as well as the outside. You are in a state of crisis and the worst thing you can do is push yourself to do more or make yourself believe that things are normal. Repeating the "Serenity Prayer" every morning or posting it at your computer might also help.

> *God give me the serenity*
> *To accept the things I cannot change,*
> *The courage to change the things I can,*
> *And the wisdom to know the difference.*

Keeping a Sense of Humor

Sometimes humor is exactly what the doctor ordered. Though hard to maintain in times of crisis, a humorous outlook can do wonders for your morale and emotional well-being. When my husband and I were undergoing artificial insemination procedures, I couldn't help but imagine that my husband's sperm was being mixed in a can and shaken up like paint at the local hardware store. This image helped me relax for the procedure and later got me great laughs when sharing it with others. How about having a date night where infertility talk is off limits? Or going to the movies to see a comedy while sharing a barrel of popcorn? Give yourself permission to act like a kid for a day. Let some laughter back into your life to help you see things in a new perspective. You may begin to accept that this, too, shall pass.

ᴇᴀ Chapter Four ᴀᴇ

Establishing a Support System

For my husband, support came in the form of a men's church choir, The Cedar Lake Seven. This citadel of strength is composed of men who sing gospel music together every Wednesday night. After being together for many years, these men have built a trust and a foundation for confiding in each other. For Greg, singing gospel music with his best friends was the perfect recipe for support. He could either seek support within the music itself, revel in the comraderie, or delve in deeper by deliberately sharing his inner turmoil. Greg began to treat this group as his sanctuary, and counted on Wednesday nights to provide the support and release he needed to sustain him through the upcoming week.

STRENGTH IN NUMBERS

Going through infertility without a support system is like jumping off a sinking ship without a life raft. You still might make it to shore, but you have drastically reduced your chances of coming up in one piece. The fact is, no one said you have to go through this alone. Include others in your journey and let them help carry the weight of your load. By letting others help, you are admitting that you can't do this alone and are willing to give up some control.

What constitutes a support system? Perhaps it is a listening ear that lets you vent relentlessly. Or confiding in people who will offer validation and not judgment. Maybe it's a friend who brings over a hot meal when you've had a particularly tough day. It might also be a church-based support group or regular meetings with a professional counselor. If this kind of support doesn't sound familiar, it is important that you try to find it.

As an extrovert, it is easy for me to confide in others. It's a way to bounce my worries off others and formulate coherent thoughts out loud. Even though this came easy to me, I still had to find a support system that was respectful of my journey through infertility. Like many people, I had to learn through trial and error. I got hurt a few times by being too open with too many people too soon. Eventually, I realized I had to distinguish who could provide a sacred place for working through my problems. For me, this included a few people who had experienced or were currently experiencing infertility. It also included individuals from my church community. Though I never attended a formal infertility support group, I was able to create a support system that fit my needs. I trusted these people and believed that God was also working through them to help me. Sometimes they would say something that hit the mark as if they instinctively knew what was troubling me that day.

Introverted people might need a bit more time to feel completely comfortable confiding in others. In fact, they may be most at ease confiding in one or two loyal friends, or a counselor or pastor. Whatever the scenario, creating a support system is a way to prevent complete isolation. It can keep you from spinning into a depression caused by getting trapped in the revolving door of the stages of grief.

𝒱ARIETIES OF SUPPORT

If you aren't sure what kind of support system would be best for you, here are some suggestions:

As a Couple

Communicate with your spouse. Revealing thoughts and feelings to one another will keep you connected and help eliminate surprises. Remember, you are going through this together as well as separately. This means you not only have to work through your own issues at your own pace, you also have to be respectful of your spouse, who may be going in a different direction at a different pace. I knew a couple who had been struggling with infertility for fifteen years. When they resolved to adopt, the husband said he was ready to adopt ten years before. For them, a lot of the pressure came from not being able to persevere together as a team.

Couple with Facilitation

Talk to someone who can think objectively and widen your view of what is happening within your situation. This could be a therapist, pastor, or someone you both trust. The facilitator's role is to ask questions that jumpstart a meaningful conversation between you and your spouse.

Support Groups

Ideally, a support group specific to your situation has the potential to provide the greatest support. Most clinics specializing in infertility should be able to refer you to a group, as should most adoption agencies. Other places to check might include hospitals and churches. RESOLVE, which is a national infertility organization, should also be able to direct you to support group resources in your area. (Contact RESOLVE at 1310 Broadway, Somerville, MA 02144-1779, or call them at 617-623-0744. You might also visit their Web site: www.resolve.org.) In the setting of a support group, you are surrounded by people who can relate to your pain and suffering because they are going through it, too. In this context of shared experience, you are likely to gain insights that you wouldn't achieve any other way.

*P*RAYER

A support system provides, in essence, a venue in which one can safely give up control. Prayer is another way of seeking support by reaching toward something bigger than yourself. Some might find it rewarding to begin each day with an original or spontaneous prayer. Others might prefer prayers written by others, which can be found in prayer collections in local libraries and bookstores.

My former pastor had a standard response to every problem: "Have you asked God?" Though this answer would bother me at times, especially when I was dealing with something complex, it eventually made sense. I think my pastor was trying to tell me that God is always available, so why not ask for help directly?

Asking God for help can mean different things for different people. Some may want to simply hand things over in silence, others may want a bit more interaction. For me, it was a dialogue. I would talk to God as I would a friend, starting with this prayer:

Dear God,

The treatments proposed to us seem radical in nature.

They replace beauty and grace with impersonal medical jargon.

We struggle with the idea of conceiving our child outside of our bodies and through artificial means.

We are even offered the option of blending our genes with another in order to increase the odds.

Give us the clarity to weigh the values in our hearts against the lure of scientific advances.

Help us to visualize the family meant for us with or without the assistance of modern medicine.

I've noticed that God is especially present to me when I put my pain into words. It's as if God is waiting for me to admit certain things to myself first before becoming involved. Somehow, saying it aloud or writing it down gives it more authenticity. It's hard to take back something once it's been said in your own voice or written in your own handwriting. It creates a sense of responsibility and ownership that wasn't there before.

After admitting or confessing the problem, you may return to the basic question: "Why do I want to be a parent?" You have already considered this question, but after focusing on it with a discerning and prayerful heart, you might be surprised at what new answers come to light. It is impossible to predict what will happen if you are willing to give up some of the control and let God join the process with you, but it is likely to be a positive experience. Evaluating some fundamental questions within the context of something bigger than yourself may begin an important internal dialogue that leads to a stronger understanding of your choices.

Once you have begun an internal conversation with God, use it to begin a conversation with your spouse. Having each worked individually and with God to get to the heart of where you stand, bring this information to one another and see how you stand as a couple. You will probably agree on some things and disagree on others. The important factor is that you are each taking responsibility for your own position, and can start working from there as a couple. Try sharing parts of your internal dialogue with your spouse. What does your spouse hear you saying? What is your spouse's opinion about this? Can you expand the dialogue together?

A support group that uses prayer provides a broader forum for God to speak through others. This can happen anywhere at anytime, whether you intentionally invite God into the process or not. But if the group is open to it, it might be helpful to pray before or after a session to invite discernment and new perspectives. If some form of prayer is acceptable to everyone, find out how the individuals view God and decide on a practice that makes everyone comfortable. If some like to read Scripture aloud and others do not, it might be better to let each person pray silently in her or his own way. Another method is to allow each person to take a turn leading the group in prayer. I have a friend who prefers inclusive language and always starts the "Our Father" with "Our Creator." Others might prefer prayer that uses images from nature. Find the language that best suits your group so that everyone feels open and willing to surrender to something bigger than themselves.

❧ Chapter Five ❧

Exploring Your Options

The options seemed endless, and in many ways, they were endless. The more I learned, the more anxious I became. For this reason, it became very important that I had a medical staff that I could trust. Although my doctor was knowledgeable and came highly recommended, I was put off by his clinical approach. He had many patients who demanded his expertise, and didn't have time to get to know me as a person. Fortunately, he had a nurse practitioner on staff who provided the human touch I desperately needed. She made herself available to answer questions and seemed to truly care about her patients. I trusted her and found her presence comforting whenever I came in for a treatment or procedure. I counted on her so much that when she transferred to a different clinic, I seriously questioned my tenacity without her.

TAKING THE INITIATIVE

Experiences and expectations vary from person to person and couple to couple. What is good for one person may not be good for another. It is necessary, however, to learn what is important to you, and you need to take the initiative in gaining this awareness. You can't control whether you will conceive or not conceive, but you can control what kind of doctor and medical environment will make you the most comfortable.

Examine every option under the lens of your own unique situation. Start imagining what kind of doctor is right for you. Make a list of qualities you would like to see in your doctor, as well as in your clinic. An infertility specialist with strong credentials may be your first choice. Or a doctor you trust explicitly who keeps your well-being in mind. Whatever you decide, it's a decision that shouldn't be taken lightly.

Most clinics offer an initial infertility consultation before starting to treat you. This is a great opportunity to get a first impression of a doctor or clinic. For example, if your questions are not getting answered during the consultation, chances are they won't be answered later, either. You may be anxious and want to start treatments immediately, but take the time to determine if the doctor or clinic suit your temperament, needs, and expectations. The last thing you want is a doctor-clinic-patient relationship that increases your stress level while undergoing treatments. Gathering information in advance can help make your experience as relaxed as possible.

Another way to investigate prospective treatments or procedures is by interviewing other couples who have already experienced them. Doctors can explain medical aspects, but may not be attuned to the emotional or spiritual effects. Do what you can to get a full picture. Prepare as much as possible to eliminate any unpleasant surprises.

Educating yourself with the help of your doctor, clinic, and outside resources will help you and your spouse make informed decisions. Most procedures and treatments have a risk factor. Use the information you have gathered for your benefit. Don't take a treatment or avoid a procedure just because it worked or didn't work for someone else.

You might consider investigating holistic approaches as well. The advantage to this route is that holistic health is geared toward the whole person—physically, emotionally, and spiritually. The disadvantage is that this kind of approach can be time consuming. Ironically, however, traditional medicine often ends up having a similar timeframe when considering the various tests that generate an accurate diagnosis and treatment plan.

Afraid to take medications with considerable risk, I began to explore holistic health options. I visited with an acupuncturist to regulate my menstrual cycle. I was told to expect treatments for approximately one year. After a few sessions, I became anxious to see some progress. I didn't have the patience that was required, so I went back to my medications. Of course, the out-of-pocket expense for the acupuncture treatments was a factor as well. It was obvious that I needed things to move along at a certain pace. The time factor became my number one priority and surpassed all other criteria.

Your Infertility Mission Statement

You and your spouse may consider writing a mission statement for your infertility process. At first, you will naturally focus on the broader questions such as:

How far will we go with treatments or procedures? How much money are we willing to spend? How much time? This is a great way to keep focused and work together as a team. Things may change over time, so it's a good idea to keep checking in with one another and discussing how your mission may have changed. You might also find that certain options come up along the way that you hadn't even considered. For example, the option of selective abortion may become an issue when a couple chooses to utilize certain fertility medications. With the help of these medications, one woman I knew had nine follicles ready for insemination, which could lead to multiple viable embryos. Her husband, much to her surprise, was unwilling to consider selective abortion should the fertilization success rate prove too great. She was devastated when he insisted on canceling the cycle. Fortunately, as you and your spouse become more experienced and focused, your mission statement will begin to narrow. Eventually, it may get as specific as: "Two more inseminations and one *in vitro* procedure, and that's it!" With the help of the mission statement, your communication can become as clear and unambiguous as possible.

When my husband and I were faced with the option of taking strong fertility medications, the ones my doctor referred to as the "big guns," we had to ask ourselves some tough questions. Did we want to risk having an over-stimulated ovary? How did we feel about selective abortion? How much increased risk was I facing as someone who has a genetic link to ovarian cancer? These were difficult, but essential, questions. We tried to focus on our own situation without comparing it to others. We had to make these decisions ourselves because we would have to live with these decisions for the rest of our lives.

REACHING THE END OF ENDLESS POSSIBILITIES

Fortunately or unfortunately, infertility presents a seemingly endless list of treatment possibilities. The scope includes surrogacy, donor eggs, donor sperm, and adoption. These are all strictly personal choices, but they all require that you ask the same fundamental question: "What is in my control and what is out of my control?" If approached in this manner, making choices becomes less a matter of right or wrong and more a matter of taking responsibility. It's a matter of drawing the line between where you choose to have your role begin and where you choose to have it end.

For my husband and me, the journey led to adoption. The turning point came after we attended a seminar on *in vitro* insemination. We were at a crossroads. It would either be *in vitro* or adoption. We went to the seminar with open minds, but discovered that, for us, the procedure crossed a boundary we were not willing to cross. We chose adoption. It was an exhilarating moment. We had made a significant decision that would reroute the course of our journey and bring us closer to wholeness.

For others, the journey may lead to various advanced treatments, surrogacy, or remaining childless. I know of one couple who came to a similar crossroads. The wife was ready for adoption and the husband wanted to continue with *in vitro*. Being divided, they made a compromise to try one more round of *in vitro*. After a successful procedure followed by a textbook pregnancy, they are now the parents of twin boys.

Adoption

In our experience, adoption signified a means to an end, but still offered plenty of challenges. The physical inconveniences of infertility are eliminated but are replaced with a whole new series of unknowns including paperwork, bureaucracy, and other unforeseen choices. You are no longer dealing with the mysteries of your body and the concept of creating life. Now you are dealing with an adoption agency, possibly another country's cultural norms, a birth mother, and a child from a different lineage. Exploring adoption, like everything else, requires research and questioning. Finding an adoption agency, deciding between domestic and international adoption, and deciding on the age of the child are just a few things to consider. Attending seminars, talking with other adoptive families, and doing individual research is always a good idea.

Adoption continues to challenge your balance. Realizing what you can and cannot control is still at the heart of it. Again, you will have to create a plan for yourselves that will enable you to take an optimal role in your area of responsibility. You will need to pay attention to the grieving cycle that this new direction causes, find the best ways to take care of yourself, establish a support system that continues to hold you up, and keep yourself informed regarding all the choices available. Then, after all that, and with no energy left, you may be convinced that you have done all you can. And as many adoptive parents will testify, their adopted children were predestined to be a part of their family right from the very start.

❧ Chapter Six ❧

Moving Toward Resolution

After months of researching, filling out forms, opening up our lives to the scrutiny of social service professionals, and waiting and waiting, relief finally came in a phone call. Our social worker wanted to know if we would be interested in adopting twin infant girls from Russia. To this day, I can't find words to describe that moment. Nor can I describe the "a-ha" feeling when I first saw our daughters on videotape. Everything inside me cried: "So there you are! You've been in Russia this whole time!"

Then, when Greg and I arrived from Russia with our sleeping daughters held near to our hearts, and with a crowd of friends and supporters waiting, we knew we had come full circle. We had come to the end of a difficult chapter in our lives. We finally had the children we always wanted and were more than ready to put infertility behind us.

Since then, however, I have found that infertility doesn't necessarily come to one perfect resolution. It's more like a process of mini-resolutions—some more significant than others. In retrospect, I can see how one resolution led to the next and how parenthood was always the goal lingering in the background. For us, infertility is now a condition that is no longer all-consuming, but continues to show itself sporadically. Being reminded by my children that they didn't grow in "mommy's tummy" is part of that condition. Knowing that if we wanted to expand our family further, we would have to go back and face the same painful issues all over again is another part of that condition.

What seemed like a resolution at one time may not feel that way all the time. I once talked with a woman who said she and her husband made the decision to stay childless a long time ago. They came to this resolution because, at the time, they were having serious financial and health concerns. Now, many years later, their lives have stabilized and they are sorry that they didn't have children. For her, it has been extremely important to keep their decision in perspective. She is comforted by the realization that at the time, remaining childless was the right decision for them. She has made peace with the fact that this chapter in their lives is over and cannot be undone.

Her message is an important one. Because you find a resolution to your infertility once, this doesn't mean that you will not need resolution in the future. Prepare for the journey ahead. Be realistic about the decisions you have made thus far and the decisions you will make in the future. Know that they will further affect you as life continues to unfold in its own way and in its own time.

Nothing about infertility is a done deal. Signs of grief and loss may creep up unexpectedly. You might find yourself in a vulnerable state again and need to nurture yourself through it. You may call on your support system or choose to build a new one that is sensitive to your current needs. You may even go back to the drawing board and explore the newest advances in reproductive medicine. Whatever comes up, be ready to find balance again. Ask yourself: "What is it I can control and what is it I can't control?" Make a list, if it helps. Dust off that "Serenity Prayer" and hang it up at eye level.

After conversing with a woman via e-mail regarding her infertility, it became amazingly apparent when resolution was about to surface. Never having seen her face or heard her voice, it became detectable in her writing. She and her husband seemed to be coming out of a fog and into what, for them, was a glimmer of light. After years and years of trying every treatment and procedure available to them, they had resolved to stop treatments after three more months. After that, they were ready to discuss other alternatives. Her writing became lighter and her tone became brighter. She was proclaiming hope for the future.

Resolution is a beautiful thing. It represents acceptance, direction, and hope. It lets you move forward when you thought your life was at a permanent standstill. It offers hope when you were beginning to think there was none left. Resolution is what you've been striving for since the very beginning. Resolution, however, is as unpredictable as infertility. It can't be reached in any one particular way. Again, it comes to each of us on its own terms and in its own time. Resolution is, more than anything else, a gift.

You can't control when it will come, but remain open to its arrival. When it does come, you will have no choice but to cherish it!

The truth is, infertility will have an effect on the rest of your life. As with any crisis, your experience with infertility will leave its mark. What kind of mark it makes, however, is really up to you. You can collect wisdom along the way or let the struggle be in vain. You can choose to become stronger, wiser, and more grateful than you ever thought possible. And who knows, someday you might even view your infertility as a blessing rather than a curse. The key is to find out where you need to take responsibility and where you need to let things go. Finding this balance will not only help you get through your struggles with infertility, but will help you with all challenges that might come your way.

Other Resources from Augsburg

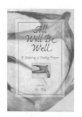

All Will be Well: A Gathering of Healing Prayers
edited by Lyn Klug
176 pages, ISBN 0-8066-3729-3

A remarkable collection of prayers expressing the hope of God's healing love.

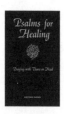

Psalms for Healing by Gretchen Person
170 pages, ISBN 0-8066-4161-4

A thoughtful collection of psalms and prayers for those who seek healing.

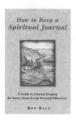

How to Keep a Spiritual Journal
by Ron Klug
144 pages, ISBN 0-8066-4357-9

A valuable resource on how to use journaling as a tool for spiritual growth.

Available wherever books are sold.
To order these books directly, contact:
1-800-328-4648 • www.augsburgfortress.org
Augsburg Fortress, Publishers
P.O. Box 1209, Minneapolis, MN 55440-1209